KSPT

Child's name: _____

Examiner: _____

Facility: _____

T0329496

INITIAL TEST

Date of testing: _____
                 (year)   (month)   (day)

Child's birthdate: _____
                 (year)   (month)   (day)

Child's Age: _____
                 (years)   (months)   (days)

Age in months: _____

PART 1 (Oral Movement)   Raw score possible=11
Raw score: _____
Standard score: _____
Percentile normals: _____
Age equivalency: _____
Percentile disordered: _____

PART 2 (Simple)   Raw score possible=63
Raw score (simple): _____
Standard score: _____
Percentile normals (simple): _____
Age equivalency : _____
Percentile disordered (simple): _____

PART 3 (Complex)   Raw score possible=81
Raw score (complex): _____
Standard score: _____
Percentile normals (complex): _____
Age equivalency: _____
Percentile disordered (complex): _____

PART 4 (Spontaneous Length)   Raw score possible=7
Raw score: _____
Standard score: _____
Percentile normals: _____
Age equivalency : _____
Percentile disordered: _____

KSPT Rating Scale/Diagnosis _____

_____

Published by [W] Wayne State University Press, Detroit, Michigan 48201.
Kaufman Speech Praxis Test for Children © 1995 by Nancy R. Kaufman. All rights reserved.

PART 1:
Oral Movement Level

Can the child execute oral movements upon command or by imitation?

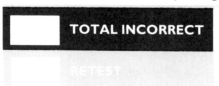

Unable to execute   Oral scanning/groping/awkward   Reduced range of movement   Unable to isolate one movement from another   Other

1   Open mouth

2   Produce voice

3   Protrude tongue

4   Lateralize tongue right

5   Lateralize tongue left

6   Alternate tongue lateralization

7   Elevate tongue to alveolar ridge

8   Spread lips

9   Pucker lips

10   Alternate spread/pucker

11   Can the child control salival pooling?   (Circle if answer is "no.")

	TOTAL INCORRECT

RETEST

TOTAL INCORRECT FOR PART 1	
RETEST	

SCORING PART I
(Oral Movement Level)

Raw score

The raw score for Part I is 11 minus the total incorrect.

$$\begin{array}{r} 11 \\ - \quad \text{(total errors)} \\ \hline \text{(Raw score)} \end{array}$$

(Retest = _____)

Age in months

If you haven't already calculated the child's age in months, see the section "Calculating Age in Months" in the KSPT Manual.

Age in months = _____   (Retest = _____)

Standard score and percentile ranking (normals)

To determine standard score as related to normals ("normal" population), use the Normative Tables in the KSPT Manual:

1. Locate the Normals tables for Part I and find the appropriate column for the child's age in months.

2. Move down the column to locate the child's raw score, then across to the standard score column.

3. To determine percentile ranking related to normals, move across again to the percentile column.

Standard score (normals) = _____   (Retest = _____)

Percentile ranking (normals) = _____   (Retest = _____)

Age equivalency

To obtain age equivalency (the age at which at least half of the "normal" children tested achieved a given score):

1. Use the age equivalency chart in the KSPT Manual and find the column for Part I of the KSPT.

2. Move down the column to locate the child's raw score.

3. Look across to the far right column to find the child's age equivalency.

Age equivalency = _____   (Retest = _____)

Standard score and percentile ranking (disordered)

To determine standard score and percentile ranking within the disordered population, use the Normative Tables in the KSPT Manual:

1. Locate the Disordered tables for Part I and find the appropriate column for the child's age in months.

2. Move down the column to locate the child's raw score, then across to the standard score and percentile ranking columns.

Standard score (disordered) = _____   (Retest = _____)

Percentile ranking (disordered) = _____ (Retest = _____)

Transfer scores from this page to the front of the test booklet.

When retesting a child after a period of treatment time, simply reuse the booklet, marking it in a different color of ink or pencil and using the "retest" scoring boxes. Repeat the steps described above to obtain a second set of scores.

PART 2:
Simple Phonemic/Syllabic Level
A. Pure Vowels (V)

Can the child produce simple isolated vowels?

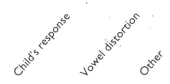

			Child's response	Vowel distortion	Other
1	/a/	(f<u>a</u>ther)			
2	/ʌ/	(m<u>u</u>ch)			
3	/u/	(b<u>oo</u>t)			
4	/i/	(<u>ea</u>t)			
5	/ɔ/	(c<u>au</u>ght)			
6	/ɛ/	(b<u>e</u>t)			
7	/ɪ/	(h<u>i</u>t)			

☐ TOTAL INCORRECT

B. Vowel to Vowel Movement (VV)

Can the child maintain the movements of two vowels together (diphthongs)?

			Child's response	Vowel distortion	Diphthong reduction	Other
1	/aɪ/	(h<u>igh</u>)				
2	/ou/	(b<u>oa</u>t)				
3	/eɪ/	(b<u>a</u>ke)				
4	/au/	(<u>ou</u>t)				
5	/ɔɪ/	(b<u>oy</u>)				

☐ TOTAL INCORRECT

TOTAL INCORRECT FOR PART I	☐
RETEST	☐

C. Simple Consonant Production (C)
Can the child produce simple isolated consonants?

		Child's response	Unable to execute	Oral scanning/groping/ awkward	Replacement/distortion/ weak target	Other
1	/m/					
2	/t/					
3	/p/					
4	/b/					
5	/h/					
6	/d/					
7	/n/					

TOTAL INCORRECT

TOTAL INCORRECT FOR PART I	
RETEST	

Circle previous consonant errors: m t p b h d n

Replacements: __ __ __ __ __ __ __

D. Reduplicated Syllables (CVCV)

Can the child imitate reduplicated syllables?

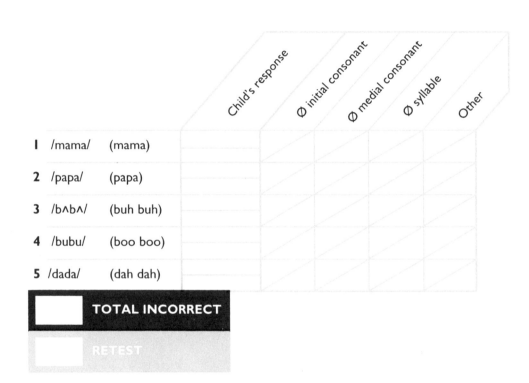

	Child's response	Ø initial consonant	Ø medial consonant	Ø syllable	Other
1 /mama/ (mama)					
2 /papa/ (papa)					
3 /bʌbʌ/ (buh buh)					
4 /bubu/ (boo boo)					
5 /dada/ (dah dah)					

TOTAL INCORRECT

RETEST

TOTAL INCORRECT FOR PART 1

RETEST

Circle previous consonant errors: m   t   p   b   h   d   n

Replacements: __ __ __ __ __ __ __

E. Consonant to Vowel Movement (CV)

Can the child maintain simple consonant production when a vowel is added?

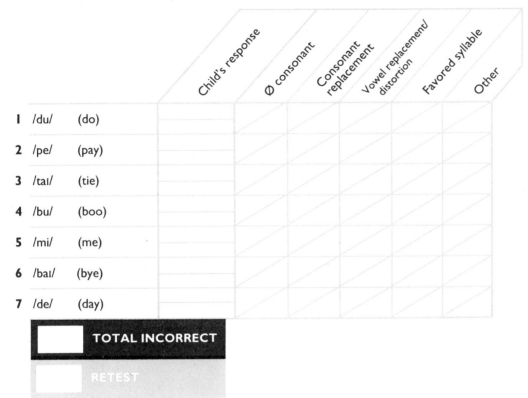

		Child's response	Ø consonant	Consonant replacement	Vowel replacement/ distortion	Favored syllable	Other
1	/du/ (do)						
2	/pe/ (pay)						
3	/taɪ/ (tie)						
4	/bu/ (boo)						
5	/mi/ (me)						
6	/baɪ/ (bye)						
7	/de/ (day)						

TOTAL INCORRECT

RETEST

F. Vowel to Consonant-Vowel Movement (VCV)

Can the child maintain two syllables with only one consonant?

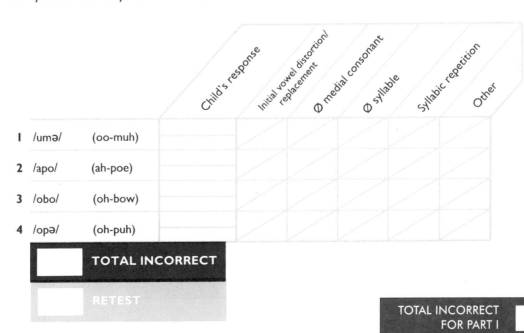

		Child's response	Initial vowel distortion/ replacement	Ø medial consonant	Ø syllable	Syllabic repetition	Other
1	/umə/ (oo-muh)						
2	/apo/ (ah-poe)						
3	/obo/ (oh-bow)						
4	/opə/ (oh-puh)						

TOTAL INCORRECT

RETEST

TOTAL INCORRECT FOR PART 1

RETEST

Circle previous consonant errors: m   t   p   b   h   d   n

Replacements: __ __ __ __ __ __ __

G. Repetitive Consonants with Vowel Change (CV₁ CV₂)

Can the child maintain two syllables when the second vowel changes?

	Child's response	Ø initial consonant	Ø medial consonant	Ø syllable	Consonant(s) replacement	Syllabic repetition	Other
1 /bʌbo/ (bubble)							
2 /mami/ (mommy)							
3 /bebi/ (baby)							
4 /pʌpi/ (puppy)							
5 /pipo/ (people)							
6 /dædi/ (daddy)							

	TOTAL INCORRECT

H. Simple Monosyllabics with Assimilation (CVC)

Can the child maintain a CVC combination when both consonants are the same?

	Child's response	Ø initial consonant	Initial consonant replacement	Ø final consonant	Final consonant replacement	Other
1 pop						
2 mom						
3 bib						
4 tot						
5 dad						

	TOTAL INCORRECT

TOTAL INCORRECT FOR PART 1	
RETEST	

Circle previous consonant errors: m   t   p   b   h   d   n

Replacements: ___   ___   ___   ___   ___   ___   ___

I. Simple Consonant Synthesis (<u>C</u>/<u>C</u>VC/CV<u>C</u>)

Can the child maintain simple initial and final consonants at the monosyllabic level?

	A				Child's response	B			Child's response	C		
	Unable to execute	Oral scanning/groping awkward	Replacement/distortion/weak target	Other		Ø initial consonant	Replacement/distortion/weak target	Other		Ø final consonant	Replacement/distortion/weak target	Other
/m/					1 <u>m</u>an				8 ho<u>m</u>e			
/t/					2 <u>t</u>op				9 kni<u>t</u>			
/p/					3 <u>p</u>in				10 ho<u>p</u>			
/b/					4 <u>b</u>oat				11 kno<u>b</u>			
/h/					5 <u>h</u>ot							
/d/					6 <u>d</u>ime				12 ma<u>d</u>			
/n/					7 <u>n</u>ap				13 bu<u>n</u>			

TOTAL INCORRECT

RETEST

TOTAL INCORRECT FOR PART I	
RETEST	

Circle previous consonant errors: m t p b h d n

Replacements: ___ ___ ___ ___ ___ ___ ___

J. Simple Bisyllabics with Consonant and Vowel Change ($C_1V_1C_2V_2$)

Can the child maintain simple syllables with consonant and vowel change?

	Child's response	Ø Initial consonant	Initial consonant replacement	Ø medial consonant	Medial consonant replacement	Ø syllable	Assimilation	Other
1 happy								
2 tummy								
3 bunny								
4 tuna								

	TOTAL INCORRECT
	RETEST

TOTAL INCORRECT FOR PART 1	
RETEST	

SCORING PART 2
(Simple Phonemic/Syllabic Level)

Raw score

To obtain the raw score, first add up all errors in Part 2 (A through J). The total possible is 63.

Then subtract the number of errors from 63.

Total errors = _____   (Retest = _____)

$$\begin{array}{r} 63 \\ - \quad \text{(total errors)} \\ \hline \text{(Raw score)} \end{array}$$

(Retest = _____)

Age in months

If you haven't already calculated the child's age in months, see the section "Calculating Age in Months" in the KSPT Manual.

Age in months = _____   (Retest = _____)

Standard score and percentile ranking (normals)

To determine standard score as related to normals ("normal" population), use the Normative Tables in the KSPT Manual:

1. Locate the Normals tables for Part 2 and find the appropriate column for the child's age in months.

2. Move down the column to locate the child's raw score, then across to the standard score column.

3. To determine percentile ranking related to normals, move across again to the percentile column.

Standard score (normals) = _____   (Retest = _____)

Percentile ranking (normals) = _____   (Retest = _____)

Age equivalency

To obtain age equivalency (the age at which at least half of the "normal" children tested achieved a given score):

1. Use the Age Equivalency Chart in the KSPT Manual and find the column for Part 2 of the KSPT.

2. Move down the column to locate the child's raw score.

3. Look across to the far right column to find the child's age equivalency.

Age equivalency = _____   (Retest = _____)

Standard score and percentile ranking (disordered)

To determine standard score and percentile ranking within the disordered population, use the Normative Tables in the KSPT Manual:

1. Locate the Disordered tables for Part 2 and find the appropriate column for the child's age in months.

2. Move down the column to locate the child's raw score, then across to the standard score and percentile ranking columns.

Standard score (disordered) = _____   (Retest = _____)

Percentile ranking (disordered) = _____ (Retest = _____)

Transfer scores from this page to the front of the test booklet.

When retesting a child after a period of treatment time, simply reuse the booklet, marking it in a different color of ink or pencil and using the "retest" scoring boxes. Repeat the steps described above to obtain a second set of scores.

Part 2 Summary Sheet

The child demonstrates the following levels of disintegration:

A. V _____   F. VCV _____

B. VV _____   G. CV_1CV_2 _____

C. C (Simple) _____   H. <u>C</u>V<u>C</u> _____

D. CVCV _____   I. <u>C</u>VC _____

E. CV _____   CV<u>C</u> _____

J. $C_1V_1C_2V_2$ _____

The child is able to produce the following simple consonants:

_____

List isolation errors:

_____

List synthesis errors:

_____

List metathetic errors (phonemes that are out of order):

_____

List epenthesis errors (phonemes that are added):

_____

The child exhibits the following consistent characteristics:

_____Open, lax vowel productions only   _____Phoneme replacements

_____Vowel distortions that are not   _____Deletion medial consonant
present in isolation
                                                  _____Syllabic repetition
_____Deletion initial consonant
                                                  _____Assimilation
_____Deletion final consonant
                                                  _____Favored sounds/syllables
_____Deletion syllables
                                                  _____Weakly targeted consonants

_____Oral scanning/groping

_____Inconsistent, off-target attempts

_____Nasal/glottal replacement

_____Verbal perseveration

_____Metathetic (reversal) errors

_____Epenthesis (addition) errors

_____Other idiosyncratic behaviors:

PART 3:
Complex Phonemic/Syllabic Level

A. Complex Consonant Production/Synthesis (<u>C</u>/<u>C</u>VC/CV<u>C</u>)

Can the child produce complex consonants? If so, can they be maintained in the initial and final contexts?

	A				Child's response	B			Child's response	C		
	Unable to execute	Oral scanning/groping/awkward	Replacement/distortion/weak target	Other		Ø initial consonant	Replacement/distortion/weak target	Other		Ø final consonant	Replacement/distortion/weak target	Other
1 /k/					16 <u>c</u>up				31 boo<u>k</u>			
2 /g/					17 <u>g</u>ame				32 bi<u>g</u>			
3 /f/					18 <u>f</u>ine				33 wol<u>f</u>			
4 /v/					19 <u>v</u>ein				34 lo<u>v</u>e			
5 /w/					20 <u>w</u>in							
6 /j/					21 <u>y</u>oung							
7 /l/					22 <u>l</u>ake				35 ba<u>ll</u>			
8 /r/					23 <u>r</u>un				36 ca<u>r</u>			
9 /s/					24 <u>s</u>un				37 bu<u>s</u>			
10 /z/					25 <u>z</u>ip				38 bu<u>zz</u>			
11 /ʃ/					26 <u>sh</u>op				39 pu<u>sh</u>			
12 /tʃ/					27 <u>ch</u>air				40 mat<u>ch</u>			
13 /dʒ/					28 <u>j</u>ump				41 ba<u>dge</u>			
14 /θ/					29 <u>th</u>ink				42 mou<u>th</u>			
15 /ð/					30 <u>th</u>em				43 ba<u>the</u>			

TOTAL INCORRECT

RETEST

TOTAL INCORRECT FOR PART 1

RETEST

Circle previous consonant errors: m t p b h d n k g f v w j l r s z ʃ tʃ dʒ θ ð

Replacements: _ _ _ _ _ _ _ _ _

Distortions: _ _ _ _ _ _ _ _

B. Blend Synthesis (<u>CC</u>VC)

Can the child maintain two consonants consecutively in context?

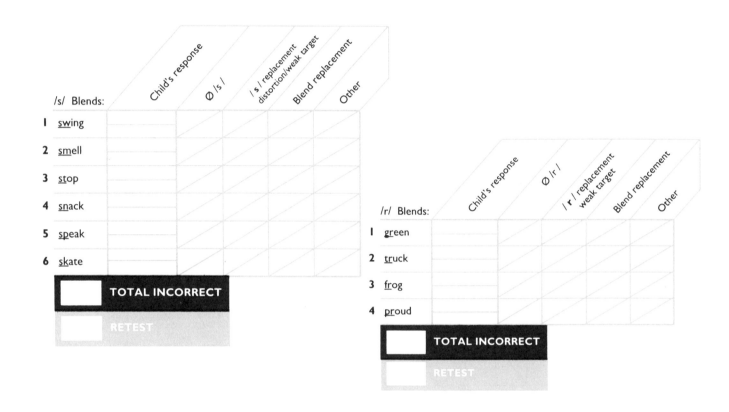

/s/ Blends:

	Child's response	Ø /s/	/s/ replacement distortion/weak target	Blend replacement	Other
1 <u>sw</u>ing					
2 <u>sm</u>ell					
3 <u>st</u>op					
4 <u>sn</u>ack					
5 <u>sp</u>eak					
6 <u>sk</u>ate					

TOTAL INCORRECT ☐

RETEST ☐

/r/ Blends:

	Child's response	Ø /r/	/r/ replacement weak target	Blend replacement	Other
1 <u>gr</u>een					
2 <u>tr</u>uck					
3 <u>fr</u>og					
4 <u>pr</u>oud					

TOTAL INCORRECT ☐

RETEST ☐

/l/ Blends:

	Child's response	Ø /l/	/l/ replacement	Blend replacement	Other
1 <u>bl</u>ack					
2 <u>cl</u>ean					
3 <u>fl</u>ag					
4 <u>sl</u>ip					
5 <u>pl</u>an					

TOTAL INCORRECT ☐

RETEST ☐

TOTAL INCORRECT FOR PART I	☐
RETEST	☐

Circle previous consonant errors: m t p b h d n k g f v w j l r s z ʃ tʃ dʒ θ ʒ

Replacements: _

Distortions: _ _ _ _ _ _ _ _

C. Front-to-Back and Back-to-Front Synthesis ($C_F VC_B / C_B VC_F$)

Can the child move from tip-alveolar to back-velar, and back-velar to tip-alveolar phonemes?

	Child's response	Fronting	Backing	Reversing	Deleting	Other
1 duck						
2 take						
3 dig						
4 get						
5 cat						
6 kid						

TOTAL INCORRECT

RETEST

TOTAL INCORRECT FOR PART I

RETEST

Circle previous consonant errors: m t p b h d n k g f v w j l r s z ∫ t∫ dȝ θ ð

Replacements: _ _ _ _ _ _ _ _ _ _ _ _ _

Distortions: _ _ _ _ _ _ _

D. Complex Bisyllabics (CVCVC)

Can the child maintain the word or previous error patterns when presented with a bisyllabic word?

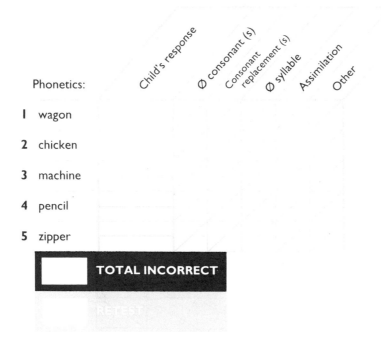

Phonetics:

1 wagon

2 chicken

3 machine

4 pencil

5 zipper

TOTAL INCORRECT

E. Polysyllabic Synthesis/Sequencing (CVCVCV)

Can the child maintain the word, the order of the syllables, or previous error patterns when presented with polysyllabic words?

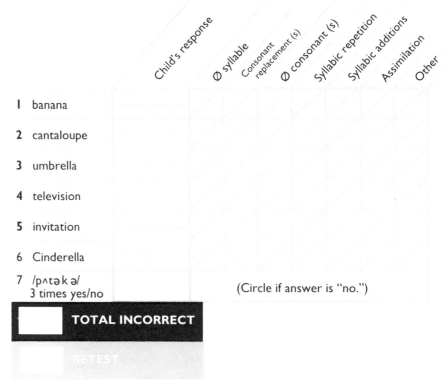

1 banana

2 cantaloupe

3 umbrella

4 television

5 invitation

6 Cinderella

7 /pʌtək ə/
   3 times yes/no   (Circle if answer is "no.")

TOTAL INCORRECT

TOTAL INCORRECT
FOR PART I

RETEST

Circle previous consonant errors: m   t   p   b   h   d   n   k   g   f   v   w   j   l   r   s   z   ʃ   tʃ   dʒ   θ   ʒ

Replacements: _

Distortions: _ _ _ _ _ _ _ _ _ _

F. Length and Complexity

Can the child maintain clarity from monosyllabic to bisyllabic to polysyllabic words?

		Child's response		Child's response		Child's response
1	win	_____	window	_____	windowsill	_____
2	bar	_____	barber	_____	barbershop	_____
3	sum	_____	summer	_____	summertime	_____
4	can	_____	cannon	_____	cannonball	_____
5	soup	_____	super	_____	superman	_____

[ ] **TOTAL INCORRECT**

TOTAL INCORRECT FOR PART I	[ ]
RETEST	[ ]

SCORING PART 3
(Complex Phonemic/Syllabic Level)

Raw score

To obtain the raw score, first add up all errors in Part 3 (A through F). The total possible is 81.

Then subtract the number of errors from 81.

Total errors = _____ (Retest = _____)

$$\begin{array}{r} 81 \\ \underline{-\quad \text{(total errors)}} \\ \text{(Raw score)} \end{array}$$

(Retest = _____)

Age in months

If you haven't already calculated the child's age in months, see the section "Calculating Age in Months" in the KSPT Manual.

Age in months = _____ (Retest = _____)

Standard score and percentile ranking (normals)

To determine standard score as related to normals ("normal" population), use the Normative Tables in the KSPT Manual.

1. Locate the Normals tables for Part 3 and find the appropriate column for the child's age in months.
2. Move down the column to locate the child's raw score, then across to the standard score column.
3. To determine percentile ranking related to normals, move across again to the percentile column.

Standard score (normals) = _____ (Retest = _____)

Percentile ranking (normals) = _____ (Retest = _____)

Age equivalency

To obtain age equivalency (the age at which at least half of the "normal" children tested achieved a given score):

1. Use the Age Equivalency Chart in the KSPT Manual and find the column for Part 3 of the KSPT.
2. Move down the column to locate the child's raw score.
3. Look across to the far right column to find the child's age equivalency.

Age equivalency = _____ (Retest = _____)

Standard score and percentile ranking (disordered)

To determine standard score and percentile ranking within the disordered population, use the Normative Tables in the KSPT Manual:

1. Locate the Disordered tables for Part 3 and find the appropriate column for the child's age in months.
2. Move down the column to locate the child's raw score, then across to the standard score and percentile ranking columns.

Standard score (disordered) = _____ (Retest = _____)

Percentile ranking (disordered) = _____ (Retest = _____)

Transfer scores form this page to the front of the test booklet.

When retesting a child after a period of treatment time, simply reuse the booklet, marking it in a different color of ink or pencil and using the "retest" scoring boxes. Repeat the steps described above to obtain a second set of scores.

Part 3 Summary Sheet

The child demonstrates disintegration at the following levels:

A. C (Complex) _____   D. CVCVC _____

    $\underline{C}$VC/CV$\underline{C}$ _____   E. CVCVCV _____

B. $\underline{CC}$VC _____   F. Length and Complexity _____

C. C_FVC_B/C_BVC_F _____

List isolation errors:

_____

List synthesis errors:

_____

List sequencing errors:

_____

The child exhibits the following consistent characteristics:

_____ phonemic deletions   _____ syllabic reversals

_____ phonemic replacements   _____ syllabic replacements

_____ phonemic additions   _____ syllabic repetitions

_____ phonemic reversals   _____ syllabic additions

_____ syllabic deletions   _____ other (specify):

PART 4:
Spontaneous Length and Complexity (Subjective Measure)

```
←————————————————————————————————→
   0     1     2     3     4     5     6     7
```

Complete <u>un</u>intelligibility   Decodable   Complete <u>in</u>telligibility

Are there more errors at this level than any other?   Yes No

Explain: _____

What phonological process patterns are noted at this level not found before? _____

_____

Are there more vowel distortions at this level?   Yes   No

Does rate of speech cause increased disintegration?   Yes   No

Are there prosodic irregularities?   Rate   Rhythm   Pitch   Intensity

Are errors felt to be motorically or linguistically based?   Motoric   Linguistic

SCORING PART 4
(Spontaneous Length and Complexity)

Raw score

The child's raw score is the number circled on the scale (0-7).

Raw score = _____　　　　　(Retest = _____)

Age in months

If you haven't already calculated the child's age in months, see the section "Calculating Age in Months" in the KSPT Manual.

Age in months = _____　　　　　(Retest = _____)

Standard score and percentile ranking (normals)

To determine the standard score and percentile ranking as related to normals, use the Normative Tables in the KSPT Manual:

1. Locate the Normals tables for Part 4 and find the appropriate column for the child's age in months.

2. Move down the column to locate the child's raw score, then across to the standard score column.

3. Move across again to the percentile column to locate percentile ranking.

Standard score (normals) = _____　　　(Retest = _____)

Percentile ranking (normals) = _____ (Retest = _____)

Age equivalency

To obtain age equivalency (the age at which at least half of the "normal" children tested achieved a given score):

1. Use the Age Equivalecy Chart in the KSPT Manual and find the column for Part 4 of the KSPT.

2. Move down the column to locate the child's raw score.

3. Look across to the far right column to find the child's age equivalency,

Age equivalency = _____　　　　(Retest =_____)

Standard score and percentile ranking (disordered)

To determine standard score and percentile ranking within the disordered population, use the Normative Tables in the KSPT Manual:

1. Locate the Disordered tables for Part 4 and find the appropriate column for the child's age in months.

2. Move down the column to locate the child's raw score, then across to the standard score and percentile ranking columns.

Standard score (disordered) = _____　　　(Retest = _____)

Percentile ranking (disordered) = _____(Retest =_____)

Transfer scores from this page to the front of the test booklet.

When retesting a child after a period of treatment time, simply reuse the booklet, marking it in a different color of ink or pencil. Repeat the steps described above to obtain a second set of scores.

KSPT Diagnostic Rating Scale Continuum

*In order to make a diagnosis of CAS the SLP should overview the key characteristics of CAS listed by CASANA (www.apraxia-kids.org)

The child's errors can be explained by:

_____ Oral structural deficit

_____ Hearing impairment

_____ Sensory-motor pathology (muscle weakness, developmental dysarthria)

_____ Auditory, perceptual, or processing challenges that include difficulty understanding the rules of the sound system (phonological disorders), resulting in mispronunciation of words

_____ Other

_____ None of the above

0.0 0.5 1.0 1.5 2.0 2.5 3.0 3.5 4.0 4.5 5.0 5.5 6.0

(EXECUTIVE)   (SECONDARY PLANNING)

0.0 ORAL-MOTOR APRAXIA (Child must be nonverbal)

_____ Difficulty moving the speech musculature upon command in the absence of oral paresis or paralysis, or oral structural deficit

_____ Difficulty initiating oral movement

_____ Oral scanning or groping during attempts to execute oral movement

1.0 VERBAL APRAXIA (EXECUTIVE)

_____ Speech disintegration in Part 2 of test at the following levels: CVCV, CV, VCV, CVC, CV_1CV_2, $C_1V_1C_2V_2$ with no significant length of utterance

_____ Single word approximations with deletions

_____ Inconsistent, off-target single words often with deletions, reversals, or repetitions

_____ Difficulty maintaining the same motor-speech pattern upon repeated trials

_____ Oral scanning/groping during imitative attempts

_____ Favored sounds, syllables, or words in place of all other sounds or words

_____ Inability to imitate motor-speech patterns of increased length or complexity over what is already shown in the speech repertoire

OTHER CHARACTERISTICS OF VERBAL APRAXIA:

_____ Accompanying oral-motor apraxia

_____ Verbal perseveration

_____ Inability to perform oral diadochokinesis

_____ Intact isolated consonant production, but breakdown at word level

_____ Vowel distortions (can be indicative of oral-motor weakness as well)

2.0   VERBAL APRAXIA (SECONDARY PLANNING)—SEVERE

_____ Disintegration on Parts 3 and 4 of test resulting in a severe speech praxis disorder marked by excessive deletions, additions, or reversals

_____ Consonant repertoire usually limited to simple consonants /m p b t d n h /

_____ Excessive replacements exist, but secondary to deletions

_____ Sound errors (distortions/weak targets) may also be present

_____ Length or complexity factors cause the system to disintegrate, contributing to unintelligibility (polysyllabic words most difficult)

_____ Inability to perform oral diadochokinesis

_____ Inconsistent, off-target attempts on certain words of increased length or complexity

_____ Better productions of single words than longer utterances

_____ Unnatural or rare phonological processes exhibited

3.0   VERBAL APRAXIA (SECONDARY PLANNING)—MODERATE

_____ Extensive replacements predominate

_____ Omissions limited to certain classes of phonemes

_____ Length of utterance and complexity continue to result in motor-speech disintegration

_____ Inability to perform oral diadochokenesis

_____ Phonological processes more consistent

_____ Better productions of single words than longer utterances

4.0   VERBAL APRAXIA (SECONDARY PLANNING)—MILD

(Note: these characteristics may overlap with phonological disorders)

_____ No deletions, additions, reversals

_____ Predictable, consistent replacements (minimal shifts in place, manner, voicing)

_____ Sound errors predominate in terms of isolated productions and thus result in synthesis errors, usually within the same class or in blends

_____ Some vulnerability with length or complexity

5.0 ARTICULATORY DISORDER

_____ Distortions, weak targets on specific phonemes, usually sibilants, or consistent articulatory inaccuracies

_____ Gliding of liquids

_____ Lateral lisps, frontal lisps, palatalization, weak /r/

6.0 NORMAL

_____ "Developmental" phoneme errors typical in age group

_____ Dialectal variations

WAYNE STATE UNIVERSITY PRESS
Detroit, Michigan 48201

1-800-WSU-READ
(313) 577-6131 FAX